How to Trim Your Hips and Shape Your Thighs

A simple exercise routine that will leave you pleasantly muscular, shapelier and fit for life!

Also by Coach Jim Everroad in Pan Books

How to Flatten Your Stomach
The sensational bestseller that's sold more than 150,000 copies

Jim Everroad's credentials include more than
fifteen years as an athlete and ten years as a
high school gymnastics coach

Lonna Mosow is a long-time fitness consultant. She is
a member of the American College of Sports Medicine

Coach Jim Everroad and Lonna Mosow

How to Trim
Your Hips and Shape
Your Thighs

Pan Books London, Sydney and Auckland

First published in Great Britain 1981 by
Pan Books Ltd, Cavaye Place, London SW10 9PG

19 18 17 16 15 14 13 12 11

© James M. Everroad and Lonna Mosow 1979

ISBN 0 330 26317 X

Printed and bound in Great Britain by
Cox & Wyman Ltd, Reading

Contents

Dedication

This one is for Sox.

Acknowledgements

Thanks to Al Gruber for his photographs, and to Dottie
Kinney for the proofreading and preliminary editing.

There are many people from the book world who have
contributed invaluable assistance and encouragement.

In particular, many thanks to Don Burkhart, Nadine
Raymer, Mike O'Leary, Bob Smith, Mike Levine and
Rick Frischman.

Special thanks to
Larry Sloan, Chuck Gates and all the other wonderful
people at Price/Stern/Sloan Publishers, Inc.

Preface

One of the many nice things about writing a best-selling book is having your publisher ask you to write another one. One *bad* thing is not knowing what to write. When *How to Flatten Your Stomach* began climbing on the bestseller lists, Price/Stern/Sloan suggested this new title: *How to Trim Your Hips And Shape Your Thighs*.

I admit to having had a terrible pot-gut, but I have always had splendid hips and thighs. Consequently, I've had very little personal experience with hip/thigh exercises.

Coaches are always looking for someone to 'do the job'. I'd have traded O. J. Simpson, Nadia Comaneci and Chris Lloyd for Lonna Mosow. Lonna knows how to trim hips and shape thighs.

A long-time fitness consultant, Lonna has developed exercise programmes for private schools, businesses, community education programmes, and modelling schools. Her programmes have been adopted by health clubs throughout the nation, and she has been a newspaper exercise columnist. For the last eight years, she has had her own highly successful TV fitness show in Minneapolis/St Paul, USA.

Lonna's personal experience with exercise includes jogging, which she began long before it became the 'in' thing. She has experimented with many exercise programmes including a five-year experiment with weight training.

She has her American national certification as a riding instructor, and much of her education and theory in animal mechanics and physiology is applicable to and useful in understanding human movement.

She is a member of the American College of Sports Medicine, and is the model for the pictures in this book. I am pleased to introduce Lonna Mosow, captain of my team, who wrote the introduction on the following page.

Coach Jim Everroad
Columbus, Indiana, USA
May, 1979

Introduction

I set out to be a ballerina – but then, doesn't every young girl? Instead, I turned out to be a physical culturist – a specialist in refining and tuning up bodies. It all began with my own body.

Working my way into the working world demanded at least four years of college, which developed my mind but left my body badly misshapen and spongy, particularly after my years of dedication to the dance. Using my knowledge and experience of body dynamics and mechanics, together with a sense of 'rightness' about kinetics, I set out to reshape my body. Later, pleased with the results – a tight, leaner, and toughened body – I refined the programme I call the *Figure Fitness Method*. It is an efficient, energetic, and effective workout which really does work. Since dancing can bring about a higher degree of muscularity than is considered attractive by most women, it was necessary to plan an exercise routine that would leave one pleasantly muscular, yet shapelier and more fit for life. All too often, the fear of overdevelopment – not to mention the fear of doing something 'wrong' – can squelch a woman's (or a man's) good intentions for body improvement.

Having shared my exercise methods with TV audiences for many years, I found the need to test the system with face-to-face instruction. For the last twelve years I have taught the *Figure Fitness Method* of exercise. Three years ago, these teaching activities led to the opening of my own studio.

The exercises I have put together here with Jim Everroad are a portion of the total *Figure Fitness Method* and have been tested and proven effective by hundreds of my students.

'Trimming our hips and shaping our thighs' will no doubt keep us – both men and women – preoccupied for a lifetime, but I hope this book will leave less to be preoccupied about! I am only one example of the success of this programme and I am happy to share these results with my students, and now, my readers.

It can be done!

Lonna Mosow
Minneapolis, Minn., USA
April, 1979

What you can do about your hips and thighs

Appearance

Women

With a placing of hands on the general hip area you say, in a fatalistic tone, 'these hips . . . what can I do about them?'

We can't tell each person how much she can improve her hips and thighs, but we can guarantee that you don't have to settle for what nature dealt you!

Improvement? Of course, it's possible, but you'll never know to what extent until you make the initial effort. The rewards can be as plentiful as the hips.

We refer to the hips as that area below the waistline that curves and bends outward and downward forming what we label 'the shelf', the hip and leg 'pones' (pone is defined as a 'pocket' of fat), and the buttocks. So, we can talk about the upper hip, the lower hip (which includes the thigh) and the outerline of symmetry (the 'fault line'). To understand the immensity of our problem, we need more than a look in a mirror. We must realize *why* we carry our excess baggage in this area.

Since we are more predisposed to carrying our body's fat stores in the general hip and thigh area, we must realize that excess fat gravitates to this area. The hip area is built with more substance because of our vertical carriage and, for that reason, can accommodate additional weight without causing hardship to the rest of the body. Consider too, that because of sluggish circulation in the area, 'sludge and garbage' aren't transported from it readily. These large muscle masses, while used in day-to-day activities, aren't taxed nearly enough to keep them in line with the rest of the body's proportions.

With our problems highly visible, and perhaps better understood, we can go about re-sculpting our hips and thighs. But it takes industrious effort to put in motion all the essential muscle groups, and to create an energy deficit to eliminate the fat stores that contribute to the hips' proportions. The programme in this book represents a proven routine that will yield a feminine and more symmetrical shape without the over-development of muscles. A soft, long, and lean line will be the result.

Men

Few men engage in physical activity which involves stretching to *improve a muscle*. Football, like most other men's sports, tends to shorten the muscles and tendons and to increase muscle size. The only reason men stretch during these sports is to loosen some specific tendons and ligaments for the purpose of avoiding injuries. Men usually think of muscular improvement as muscle building until they stop playing football or other sports and buy a new pair of trousers.

It is then that they decide to slim their thighs. Since their only exercise frame of reference is in those activities which tend to increase muscle size, they are lost. The programme in this book can help them reduce the size of their thighs.

Health

Anatomy and physiology

This programme is designed to stretch and contract many muscles. Some of the muscles are attached to the ridges of the hip bones, and to other points on the front, sides and back of the hip bones. With a few exceptions, they then extend down the legs. Some are attached again to the front, sides and back of the upper legs. Others extend further down, attaching to the knee-caps, and to the front and back of the lower legs.

The easiest muscle to identify is the gluteus maximus. Its two parts form the buttocks. You can touch your quadriceps muscle along the entire front and outer sides of your upper legs. You can also feel the quadriceps on the lower front towards the inner sides of the upper legs. Your hamstrings can be touched from below the buttocks to the tops of the calf muscles. The adductor magnus muscle can be felt next to the hamstrings on the inner rear of the upper legs.

Many of these muscles are difficult to identify, but they can be located by touch. The tensor fasciae latae and gluteus minimus can be touched just in front of, and above, the joint of the thigh bone and the hip. The rectus femoris, pectineus, adductor longus, and gracilis muscles can be felt on the front of each upper leg near the pubic area.

Some of these muscles cannot be seen or felt. These include the iliacus, sartorius, gluteus medius, adductor brevis, popliteus, and six deep muscles for rotating the leg outwards.

The muscles worked in this programme include a high percentage of the total muscle mass of your body. We have briefly mentioned twenty-two different muscles located on each side. In addition, each muscle is made up of many fibres, which range in size from a fraction of a centimetre to 460 centimetres. They are very thin; no more than 0·016 millimetres thick. When a muscle works, some or all of its fibres contract, becoming shorter.

Muscle contractions will build tone, strength, and endurance in the muscles to combat flabbiness and improve contour. Chemical reactions which cause, and result from, muscle contractions will utilize glycogen, fat, and other nutrients stored in the muscles. (Exercise is the most efficient method of breaking down *fat*.) Utilization, rather than excessive storage of these nutrients, will produce a slimming effect.

The fibres can also be stretched beyond their normal length. The muscles' tendons, which attach the muscles to the bones, can be stretched with the muscle fibres. Stretching the fibres and tendons increases flexibility at the joints, and will strengthen the fibres through their entire range of motion. Stretching will tend to slim the muscle fibres.

This programme is *not* designed to increase the size of muscles. (Exercises in which the muscles work against heavy resistance are necessary to develop size.) It is, rather, a programme of prolonged, continuous movement, which emphasizes stretching and mild muscle contractions.

Direct functions

Some of the muscles of this programme bend the knee, and some straighten it. Others move the thigh bone at the hip joint. A few cause movements at both the knee and hip joints. The thigh bones (upper legs) can be moved apart and together, and forwards and backwards. Also, the thigh bones can be rotated inwards and outwards. Combinations of these movements can be executed by coordinated effort of the different muscles. This programme is designed for the performance of a large variety of these movements.

The hip/thigh muscles also act directly to pump blood from the feet and lower extremities, through veins, back to the heart. Blood can flow through veins towards the heart, but not away from it, since the valves open only in one direction. When the muscles contract, they squeeze the veins, forcing blood through the veins' valves. The pumping action of the muscles is especially important in the legs, since blood pressure in the veins of the legs tends to be higher than in the veins of the upper body. Without sufficient pumping action from the muscles, the pressure in the veins will become too high. Inactivity of these muscles is one of the causes of a very common problem: varicose veins.

Varicose veins

If the blood pressure in a vein increases too much, the vein will become too large for its valves. Then the valves fail to keep blood moving towards the heart, and blood becomes pooled in the veins. This condition is known as varicose veins.

The most common varicose veins are the great and small saphenous veins. The small saphenous veins run from the outside of each foot up the back of the calves. The great saphenous vein runs from the inside of each foot, up the inside of the legs, towards the pubic area. These veins and their tributaries are located very close to the surface, and they are easily seen when they become varicose.

The blood pressure in the veins can become too high for several reasons, including excessive weight, pregnancy, and above-average height. The simplest method of keeping the blood pressure at its proper level is to use the muscles surrounding the veins. This book's programme effectively uses those muscles which pump blood through the saphenous veins and their tributaries. The programme also builds and maintains tone in these muscles, making the venous pump more efficient.

Varicose veins are a source of worry and concern among pregnant women. Use of this programme prior to pregnancy will help you avoid varicose veins. We do not advise *beginning* this programme *after* you have become pregnant. If you have been using this programme *prior* to pregnancy, you can continue it during pregnancy, *but do so only with your doctor's advice and approval*.

Controlling your physiology

This is a high performance fitness programme. Using it allows you to direct and control much of your body's physiology. Exercise provides you with maximum direction and control over what is happening inside your body, and it is the only natural way to achieve this. Let's be specific about what you can control and direct.

Blood carries oxygen and other nutrients to the muscles and other tissues. The flow of blood to the muscles increases dramatically during exercise because the exercising muscles need more nutrients due to their increased activity. At rest, only fifteen to twenty per cent of your body's total blood flow goes to your muscles. The extent to which you can direct your body's physiology is illustrated by the following: *During heavy exercise the blood flow to the muscles can increase more than fifteen-fold.* This means that in heavy exercise there is up to three times more blood pumped to the *exercising muscles* than is pumped throughout the *entire body* at rest.

Your heart pumps whatever amount of blood flows into it, within physiologic limits, and more blood flows into it during exercise. The more blood that flows into it, the more your heart's muscle fibres stretch. The more the fibres stretch, the harder they contract. The harder the heart contracts, the more blood it pumps.

Your heart also beats faster during exercise, increasing the amount of blood it pumps. The increased heart beat and the increased amount of blood pumped with each contraction cause an astonishing increase in the total amount of blood pumped by the heart. In fact, the heart could pump the equivalent of every drop of blood in your body as quickly as *every ten to twelve seconds* during heavy exercise.

This increased output of blood by the heart and the increased flow of blood to the muscles provide many positive results. The heart and exercised muscles will be stronger and have more endurance. There will be an increased number of blood vessels to nourish the heart and the exercised muscles, and the metabolism in the muscles will increase, burning many extra calories. I hope the enormous extent to which you can control and direct this activity has been sufficiently discussed. Exercise is the *only* natural way to utilize this control.

Cardiovascular fitness

People are said to have, or lack, cardiovascular fitness according to several different formulas. One simple formula is whether or not you can maintain a pulse rate of 120 beats per minute, for fifteen to twenty consecutive minutes. If you can do this four or five times a week, in reasonable comfort, you are cardiovascularly fit, according to this definition. Being able to do this demonstrates efficiency in the lungs, and strength and efficiency in the heart and circulatory system. The hip/thigh programme can help you achieve and maintain cardiovascular fitness.

Your understanding of cardiovascular fitness can be increased by reading any number of good, current books. One we would suggest is *The Aerobics Way*, by Dr Kenneth Cooper.

Running is also excellent for cardiovascular fitness. If you are a runner (jogger), these exercises are especially worthwhile for you. Most runners know that the muscles and tendons in the hips, knees and ankles must be stretched to avoid problems that can be caused by running. These problems include injuries to the joints, muscles and tendons, and postural problems. This programme does an excellent job of keeping the tendons and muscles stretched, and the joints flexible. It is also a good workout for those days when you do not run.

For those wanting more 'mileage' from the hip/thigh exercise plan, we would advise a running/walking programme. You can build tremendous endurance in your hip and thigh muscles by running fifteen to twenty minutes three or four times a week. However, it is important that you build to this level slowly over a long period of time, starting out by walking briskly at the outset.

Follow the hip/thigh programme for a couple of weeks before starting to run/walk. This will prime your muscles, heart, and lungs and mobilize underactive joints, tendons and ligaments. Continue to use these exercises *with* a running programme. We would *not* advise *only* running if you are truly concerned about your hips and thighs.

Obesity

Lack of exercise is a major cause of obesity, mainly because it is too easy for most people to ingest more calories than they burn – unless they exercise. Your 'resting metabolism' requires *so few calories* that it takes *very little* food to provide too many. As we know, only too well, the excess calories are stored as fat.

The second reason is less obvious and more important. It has recently been discovered that areas of the brain's hypothalamus actually control a person's appetite and satiety. Experiments by Dr Jean Mayer, one of the world's foremost nutrition experts, have shown that these areas do not function properly without sufficient exercise. At very low levels of activity appetite does not decline sufficiently and you will take in more calories than are burned. With enough exercise, these mechanisms will remind you to eat when you *need* more calories. The mechanisms will also remind you to stop eating when you've had enough.

Summary

There are, then, at least eight reasons for using this programme to trim your hips and shape your thighs:

1. It will improve your appearance.

2. It will increase the tone, endurance, and strength of your hip/thigh muscles.

3. It will stretch your tendons, ligaments, and muscles, increasing the flexibility and mobility of your joints.

4. It will improve the venous pump, thereby helping you to avoid varicose veins.

5. It will allow you to control much of your body's physiology by directing the activity of your heart.

6. It will help you build and maintain cardiovascular fitness.

7. It will condition you well for the beginning of a running programme, and it is an excellent supplement to a running programme.

8. It will help you overcome obesity.

About the programme

Although some of the more traditional exercises have been included here, it takes somewhat 'more creative' exercise to engage in motion all the essential muscle groups. Using all of the essential muscle groups will bring about enough energy deficit to eliminate the fat stores that contribute to the hips' generosity.

The selection and combination of exercises in this programme were based on the following factors:

Simplicity – Simple motions are highly effective because they are less likely to be mistreated and will, therefore, be executed with precision and accuracy. Many of us who have never engaged in exercise or sports have little awareness of the body's potential for motion.

Efficiency – Efficient exercises are those that force as many muscle areas as possible into motion at the same time. This provides contouring and also places demands on the body for additional expenditure of energy.

Fringe benefits – These exercises affect the specific muscle area for contour and help improve flexibility, joint mobility, muscular endurance, strength, and tone, all of which will yield a better-proportioned figure. It also provides a greater ability to move, which is the cornerstone of effective exercising.

Anti-stress – These exercises 'stress' the hips and thighs in a positive way, while avoiding stress to the most vulnerable area of the body, the spine. We refer to this as positive and negative stress, or 'stress without stress!'

Teaming – All the exercises complement and reinforce each other's effects, but without unnecessary duplication.

Sequencing – Apart from the above exercise factors, the success of this programme depends not only on the execution of each exercise, but also on its position in the sequence. *The programme should be followed exactly as presented, without deletions*. It is structured so that the first set of exercises is done at the 'standing level'. Each exercise relates to the next one without unnecessary shifting of position. The second set is at the 'support level', with each exercise designed to flow conveniently to the next one. The third set is at the 'floor level', and completed in one of two methods (see page 29). The fourth level, 'peak level', completes the cycle of exercises and returns you to the initial standing position.

Disciplining

Using a tested and proven exercise programme is one thing; making it work is another. This exercise programme will be as effective as you make it. In shaping hips and trimming thighs, you must first lay the foundation for success. You can do this by disciplining yourself. It will assure you of results and will help you maintain these results. Prepare for your programme by doing the following:

1. Set up a specific area for your exercises. Your mini-gym should be at a comfortable temperature and should allow enough space for broad-range kicks and leg swings. The general atmosphere should be pleasant. Avoid an area of your home that suggests work.

2. Choose a time of day that is not likely to be interrupted by children, pets, phone calls or doorbells. All these provide easy excuses for 'I'll do it later!' Finding a perfect time will take some experimenting because – apart from interruptions – your energy level at certain times of the day may not permit you to exercise at your peak. However, exercising during an 'energy low' may prove acceptable for certain people. You must discover this for yourself. Once you have found a time that fits your schedule and your energy level, reserve that time and organize your day around it.

3. Choose an exercise outfit that feels good on you and reserve it just for your exercise sessions. The mere slipping on of this uniform will prepare you psychologically for your session. Informal clothing is best – pyjamas, shorts, leotards, old sweatshirt, bathing suit – anything that will help put you in the right mood.

4. You should also include a special prop, such as a favourite beach towel to lie on, music, or mirrors. Also, because some of the exercises rely only on a chair, be sure to use the *same* chair for each of your sessions.

5. Avoid waiting for your life style to 'right' itself so that you can start this programme. Because holidays, social events, children's activities, and work commitments are unlikely to change, start your programme to fit into the 'right now!' What better time to begin your exercise programme than on a holiday. Too many 'starts' and 'finishes' will certainly finish your programme before you begin to experience any results. Interruptions in your exercise schedule will set the pattern for future interruptions, in addition to making the programme ineffective.

Organize your workout days in one of three ways:

1. Discipline yourself to exercise on an every-other-day schedule, filling in the 'off' days with constructive recreation or fitness activities — walking, jogging, biking, swimming, handball, tennis, etc. If you exercise every other day, you should hold on to one schedule for a two-week period.

2. Or, discipline yourself to exercise daily if you have no other means for working your muscles, joints, tendons, and ligaments. During your seven-day week, be sure to schedule no less than four exercise sessions.

3. Structure your hip and thigh programme to *reinforce* your other daily fitness activities. Many of the hip/thigh exercises have a built-in stretch for improving your flexibility either *before* or *after* a run. Because of the stimulation of blood flow and increased joint mobility, these exercises can be teamed with any other exercise activities to accelerate their enjoyment and expected results.

How to use this programme

Let's start!

To insure yourself of the shapeliest hips and trimmest thighs, practise these exercise principles:

1. *Standing exercises* – In order for the body to be free to move from all joint areas, and in order to avoid excessive stress on the lower back, an *anti-gravity* posture should be maintained throughout any exercises done from a standing position. To achieve this anti-gravity posture, when standing on one leg, be sure to 'lift up' from the small of the back and rib cage. At the same time, avoid stiffening the body, since this will cause a locking of all joint areas, which must be at ease in order to move through their complete range of motion.

2. *Floor level exercises* – While lying on your side, keep a straight line from your shoulders through your hips and legs so that your spine will be in good alignment. Your forward arm can be a source of support, so rely on it. When lying on your back, place your hands beneath your hips so that you add support to your lower back. Be aware of your spine, always maintaining good body alignment while doing exercises on the floor.

3. *Breathing and pace* – Your exercise pace is regulated in part by even, rhythmic breathing and by the amount of time needed to complete a repetition (rep). Conscious inhaling and exhaling, while in motion, will help your exercise pace. It is important to set your pace at a comfortable level right from the start, since that pace should be maintained consistently throughout the exercises. All too often, as you speed up an exercise, the shortened motion will yield considerably lessened results.

There are suggested *Time guides* listed with each exercise, to serve as a guide in pacing. The guides are suggested times for completing ten reps. Only when you are completely familiar with the exercises, and have made considerable progress with the programme, should the guides be applied. The guides are set up so you will perform the programme energetically. Do not lower the pace as you increase your repetitions above ten.

4. *Perpetual motion* – For your programme to work, *you* must work! Once you are familiar with each of the exercises, keep moving – without breaks or rest periods – from one repetition to another, from one exercise to another. Maintaining perpetual motion will cause your programme to have a cardiovascular effect and will place more demands on your body. A better body and better fitness will be the result.

5. *Attitude* – A certain mental awareness should accompany the physical aspect of the programme – awareness of using certain muscles, how a movement feels, how to isolate a given muscle or breath while kicking a leg, or how to relax some

muscles while working others. Your mental awareness will help your mind and muscles work together for maximum results.

First study the exercise descriptions, practising the movements as you progress. Learn to perform each of the exercises and begin to apply the exercise principles already discussed. Learn to recognize them simply by looking at the pictures. This will take some time, but be patient and conscientious about learning the exercises correctly; the programme is well worth it.

The number of repetitions you can do and the length of time you can continuously exercise will vary depending on your starting fitness level. Some muscles are stronger at the outset and will enable you to accommodate more repetitions per exercise. Although each exercise *must be included*, you will not necessarily repeat each exercise the same number of times. Some muscles are more responsive and, therefore, will respond faster than others, so expect *non-uniformity* in the beginning. 'Lazy' muscles will take more time and effort and your persistence with these stubborn areas will pay off.

Repeat each exercise as many times as you can while still maintaining a 'clean' motion. As you feel muscles tiring during an exercise, or motions becoming 'slurred', hurried or sloppy, go on to the next exercise. This will keep you in motion, but allow tired muscles to rejuvenate while others continue to work. As a rule of thumb, begin each of the exercises with ten repetitions. If any of the exercises prove to be overly difficult, do fewer until the muscles strengthen.

As you progress, you will become familiar with each exercise and its position in the sequence. At the same time, your fitness level for doing the exercises will improve, and you can increase your repetitions.

The standing level exercises are numbers 2 and 3; the support level exercises are numbers 4 to 9b; the floor level exercises are numbers 10 to 14; and the peak level exercises are numbers 15a and 15b. You will notice that the programme is a complete cycle, starting and ending in the standing position.

When you are performing twenty repetitions of every exercise with good form (smoothness, coordination, and proper pace), try sequencing the floor level as follows:

Instead of completing twenty repetitions (reps) of each floor level exercise on both sides of your body first, complete *each* floor level exercise at least ten times using the *same* leg in sequence. Then, when you have completed the floor level sequence with one leg, repeat it with the other leg.

It is a good idea to see your doctor before beginning any exercise programme: it is an even better idea to see him if you are planning *not* to start one.

Excellent exercises for trimming the hips and shaping the thighs

1 Be sure you have read the first three sections of this book before beginning these exercises. Your success with this programme will be in direct proportion to your understanding of its value and its proper use.

2 Stand, feet one metre apart, knees at ease (straight, but not locked), arms straight overhead, elbows straight, palms towards ceiling, with fingers interlocked. Keep your heels on the ground, but feel most of your weight on the balls of your feet. Stretch upwards, lifting the rib cage. Then, with your upper body, do a free-flowing fall forwards and down while *deeply bending your knees*. Reach back through the legs as far as possible, emphasizing stretch in the hip and thigh area (pictured). Immediately swing the upper body back up to the starting position, and avoid arching the back. This is 1 repetition (rep).

This exercise should and will become smoother and more rapid with practice. Time guide: 15 seconds.

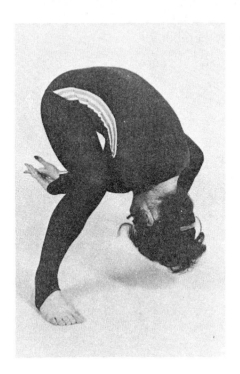

3 Stand, feet one metre apart, knees at ease. Bend *deeply* forward at the waist, letting your head and upper body hang down. Stay relaxed in the upper body. Feel most of your weight on the balls of your feet (heels on floor) and stay relaxed with no stress in your back. Stretch your arms sideways, parallel to the floor, elbows straight. Now you are in the starting position. Rotate your shoulders so the right shoulder moves across the front of your body to the left, and avoid moving your upper body sideways from the waist to the left. As you rotate your shoulders, reach to the left with the right hand, and attempt to touch the floor on the left side of your left foot for 1 rep. Avoid lifting your head and shoulders as you immediately return *through* the starting position to repeat with the left shoulder and hand moving to the right (pictured) for rep number 2.

Continue with no pause at the starting position until you have finished your reps. Do the reps rapidly, with lots of momentum, and feel stretch in your inner thighs. Time guide: 6 seconds.

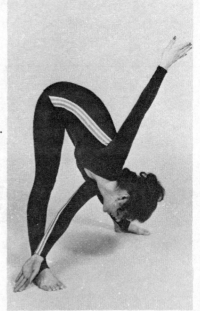

4 Stand behind a chair. Stand close to it, facing the back of it. Place both hands on top of the chair's back, but avoid leaning on it. Spread your legs almost as wide as possible (more than one metre at least), knees and toes pointed directly out to your sides, knees at ease. Bend your knees and lower your body as far as possible (pictured), then return to starting position for 1 rep.

Imagine a brick wall standing very close in front of you. Avoid scraping the wall with the knees, head, and chest as you do the exercise. Time guide: 14 seconds.

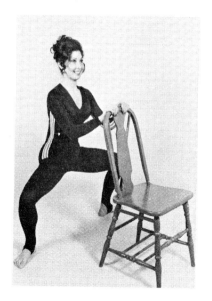

5 Stay down without returning to starting position after exercise 4. Stay as low as possible and remember the brick wall in front of you. 'Slide' your hips and upper body to the left, without moving either foot, increasing the bend in your left knee, until your right knee is straight and locked and most of your weight is on your left foot, for 1 rep (pictured). Remain *low* and immediately slide back to the right, until the left leg is straight, with knee locked, for rep number 2. Move continuously, with no pause at starting until you have finished your reps. Time guide: 10 seconds.

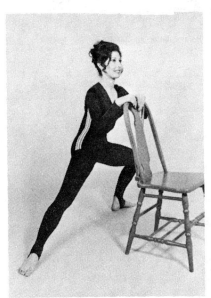

6   Stay close to the chair, not leaning on it (use it for balance only), stand straight, feet together. Feel weight on the balls of your feet (heels on floor), knees at ease. Kick one leg sideways, keeping the foot *flat*, and the *knee and toes pointed forward*. Avoid letting the upper body lean in the opposite direction of the kick. Don't scrape the brick wall with your knee or thigh. Kick as high as possible, without leaning the upper body in any direction (pictured), and while keeping the toes pointed forward (there is no brick wall in front of your toes).

Do rapid repeats without pausing at the starting position until you are finished with your reps. Time guide: 7 seconds. This is the *kwik kick*. Do the same number of reps with the other leg.

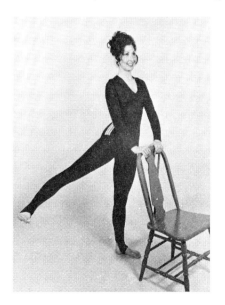

7 Stand facing either the right or left side of the chair, about one metre away from it. Bend forward at the waist and grip the *front* of the chair seat with one hand, keeping the elbow straight, shoulder over the hand. Place your other hand and elbow (forearm) on top of the chair's back. Your hips should be leaning slightly over your feet towards the chair. Rest enough body weight on the chair so you feel no stress on your lower back. Keep the foot of one leg *flat* and *kick* that leg back and up as high as possible, while avoiding letting your hip turn upwards/outwards during the kick (pictured). Immediately return the leg to starting position for 1 rep. Do rapid repeats without pausing at the starting position until you are finished with the exercise. Time guide: 13 seconds. Do the same number of reps with the other leg.

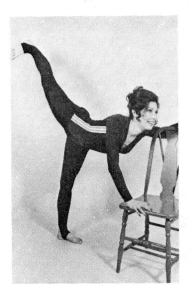

8 Stand straight, still facing the side of the chair, and hold the top of the chair's back with the hand closest to it. Raise the opposite knee close to your chest, attempting to hold your balance on one foot. Grab either your ankle or instep and pull it in tight, and you are now in the starting position. Keep your ankle in tight and move your knee downwards until the knee is pointed directly towards the floor. Lean forward and pull the leg up as high as possible in back. At the same time you are pulling your leg up in back, push your ankle hard against your hand straightening the knee as much as possible. Emphasize getting the leg high, pushing hard against the hand with your ankle, and your elbow will be straight at the peak of the movement (pictured). *Try to maintain your balance on one foot, using the chair only to help with the balance.* After reaching the peak of the movement, return immediately to the starting position for 1 rep. No time guide. Emphasize balance, stretch, and coordination. Do the same number of reps with the other leg.

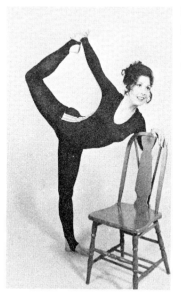

9a Stand at least one metre in front of the chair. Face the chair, spread your legs almost as wide as possible (more than one metre, in any case), keep your feet pointed forward, legs straight, knees at ease. Bend forward and place both forearms on the chair seat, elbows bent and palms and elbows down on the chair seat, shoulders over your elbows. Your hips should not lean to the front or back of your feet, so adjust your distance from the chair accordingly. Feel comfortable. Move your hips to the right, pointing your right knee to the right, and letting your right knee bend deeply. During the movement the right foot should pivot on the heel so the toes point to the right, and you should let the left foot roll on to its right side, keeping the left leg straight. Move steadily for a long stretch, bending the knee deeply (pictured), for 1 rep. Immediately return *through* starting position, and repeat to the left, pivoting on the left heel so the toes point to the left, and letting the right foot roll on to its left side for rep number 2. Time guide: 13 seconds.

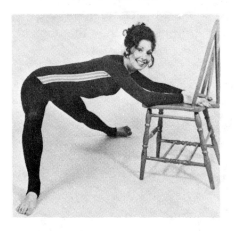

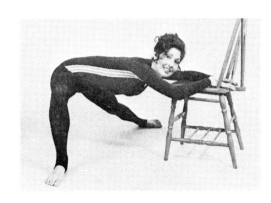

9b After your last rep of 9a stay in the deep knee bend position, and this is your starting position for exercise 9b. You will find you can concentrate and bend the knee further when you do not move immediately back in the other direction. With a relaxed, easy movement, bend the knee *deeper* (pictured), emphasizing a smooth stretch. Return *only* to the deep knee bend starting position, without straightening the knee for 1 rep. Do your reps continuously, but avoid bouncing, emphasizing stretch, not speed. Make certain that you complete all your reps on one side before starting on the other side. Time guide: 13 seconds.

10a Lie on your back, hands under the buttocks, palms on floor, one leg straight with the foot flat (toes pointed at the ceiling), the other knee bent with the foot flat on the floor. Keep the leg straight and kick it up as far as possible in one quick, smooth motion (pictured). Avoid moving the bent knee, keeping the foot flat on the floor during the movement to 'anchor' the exercise. Immediately return to starting position for 1 rep. Do your reps continuously without pausing at the starting position. Time guide: 13 seconds.

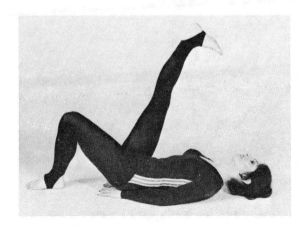

10b   Same starting position as 10a. Again kick the leg straight up. When you have kicked as high as possible, your leg will 'bounce' slightly back towards the floor. Do not let it return to starting position, but instead do an immediate second kick, still keeping the leg straight, and bring it as close to the upper body as possible (pictured). Immediately return to starting position as in 10a for 1 rep.

Do your reps continuously without pausing at the starting position. Time guide: 19 seconds.

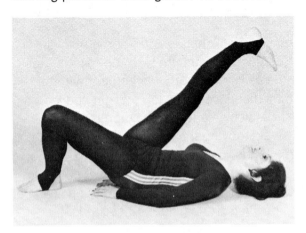

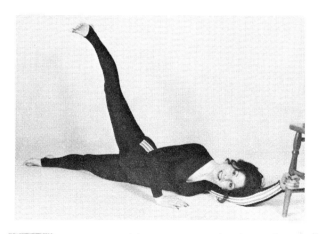

11a Lie on one side, arm stretched overhead, hand grasping a leg of the chair for support, head resting on the bottom arm and shoulder, palm of the top hand on the floor in front of your chest, elbow bent, legs straight and together, top foot *flat* with toes pointed forward. Viewed from the top, there should be a straight line from the grip hand to the shoulder to the hip to the foot. A line from the top shoulder to the bottom shoulder should run straight down (perpendicular) to the floor. Also, a line through both hips should run straight down to the floor. Raise the top leg as high as possible, keeping the toes pointed forward and foot *flat* (pictured). Avoid letting the toes turn upwards, or moving the foot to the front or back during the movement. Lower the leg completely for 1 rep. Emphasize speed in the leg raise, and do your reps continuously without pausing at the starting position. Time guide: 12 seconds.

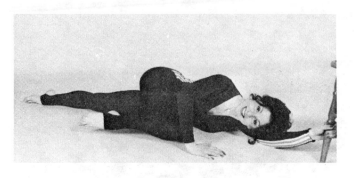

11b Begin immediately after your last rep of 11a. Pull your top knee forcefully along the floor, 'power driving' it as close to the chest as possible. Bend the knee completely as it comes towards the chest (pictured). Immediately return along the same path to the starting position. Without pausing, raise and lower the leg as in 11a, alternating the two motions for 1 rep.
Time guide: 22 seconds.

12 Lie on your side as in 11a and b (on your left side). Roll slightly on to your left buttock, while raising your leg forward and up, until it is pointed straight up from the floor (picture A). This is your starting position. Then immediately bend the knee while again rolling on to the left side (picture B), continue rolling foward almost on to your stomach, keeping the knee bent, while

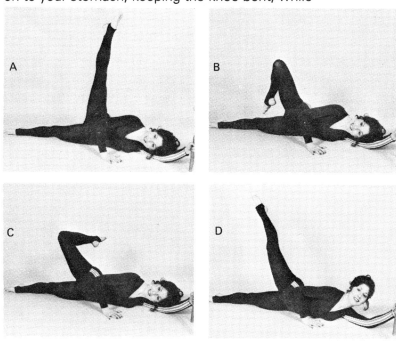

moving the leg down and backwards (picture C), then straighten the knee bringing the leg up and back as high as possible (picture D). From this position, again bend the knee, rolling back on to your left side, while moving the leg down and forward; continue rolling back on to your left buttock, while raising the leg forward and up, then straightening the knee so the leg is again in starting position (picture A). This is 1 rep. We call this exercise the *Hollywood swing*.

While you are learning this exercise, you will stop at each pictured position. Once you understand the positions, begin to move through them to make the exercise one continuous movement. To help you do so, we offer the following suggestions: Think of bending the knee while rolling, and straightening it at the end of each roll. Also, think of lowering the leg while rolling on to the side, and raising it while rolling off the side. Expect to take some time to get the coordination for this exercise. It is the most complicated exercise in the programme, but one of the most rewarding. Time guide: 22 seconds.

13 The *hip stripper*. Same position as 11a then raise your upper body and place your elbow on the floor under your shoulder, and bend your knees so both lower legs are pointed straight behind you (at a right angle). Avoid moving your legs forward at the waist, and you are in the starting position for this exercise. Relax, keep your back in a comfortable position. Keep your knee bent, and quickly raise (pictured) and lower your top leg, including the knee and foot, for 1 rep. Emphasize speed and a high leg raise.
Time guide: 10 seconds.

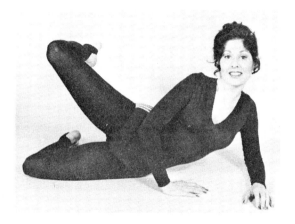

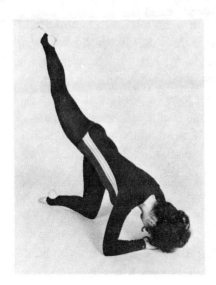

14 The *bun burner*. Start on your hands and knees (all fours), then place your elbows on the floor. Put your hands together, then lean down with your head and shoulders, and rest your head on your hands. Straighten one knee, and keep the foot on the floor to come to the starting position. Kick the straight leg back and up as high as possible (pictured). Avoid letting your leg turn outwards/upwards during the kick. Immediately lower the leg, keeping it straight for 1 rep. Avoid pausing at the starting position between reps. Do fast kicks and rapid repeats, but emphasize height in the kick. Time guide: 12 seconds.

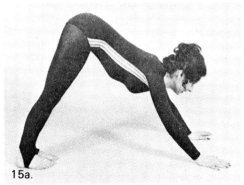

15a.

15a Start on your hands and knees (all fours), feet and knees together, with the bottom of the toes on the floor. Keep the toes and hands in place, and straighten your knees, pushing your rear up and attempting to bring your heels down until they are flat on the floor (pictured). Emphasize stretch in the back of the legs. Immediately lower to starting position for 1 rep. Avoid pausing at the starting position between reps. Time guide: 13 seconds.

15b The *knee kiss*.
After the last rep of 15a, walk your hands as far back as possible, bringing your heels down to the floor, then come to a balanced position on your feet. Knees at ease, grab the back of your ankles, and use a steady gentle pull to try to 'kiss' your knees (pictured). Hold the tightest position you can reach for a count of 10. Do only 1 rep. Stay relaxed and breathe normally.

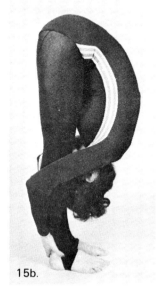

15b.

16 From the knee kiss position, spread your feet as in exercise 3, repeat exercise 3, and then repeat exercise 2 to finish your workout.

Enjoy your workouts, and let us know how you progress. You may write to Coach Jim Everroad and Lonna Mosow, c/o Price/Stern/Sloan Publishers, Inc., 410 N. La Cienega Blvd, Los Angeles, Ca. 90048, USA.